What families who are dealing with a brain tumor have to say about
Brain Tumors-Leaving the Garden of Eden

…explains the complex issues of brain tumors in a manner that the general public can understand - without 'talking down' to us… the tone is crisp and reads well… Ray G, Albany NY

Written well from the beginning… you can … see this book is not like a Physician's Desk Reference. Patty A, a survivor in NJ

I was struck by how much I did not know even though I have been researching brain mets on behalf of several friends with melanoma and breast cancer brain mets. Helen S, NY

… a roadmap through what is complicated and scary to the lay reader. The Checklist To Assess My Team & Care is empowering, challenging and clear ….and will piss off lots of doctors! … in a good way. Shira G,TV writer, CA

Inspiringly hopeful…so admirable - coming from a physician instead of an on-line bulletin board or support group. Katie C, UCLA, Los Angeles

I have wished for this book. The chapter on the Team is probably the best thing I have read on this… ever! "… successful patients not only learn how to 'work the system' but they also learn how to live in this foreign land." This book shows you how. Loice, Philadelphia, PA

You can take comfort in having Dr. Zeltzer with you during your brain tumor journey. Naomi Berkowitz, Executive Director, American Brain Tumor Association, Chicago,IL

More comments from readers who are dealing with a brain tumor and what they have to say about
Brain Tumors-Leaving the Garden of Eden

The personal e-mail comments express familiar situations I'm sure will strike a vote with all those who read the book...it connects on a personal level. Christine D, Austin, TX

A "how to" book when your world is falling apart... you're a person... not a patient or a statistic. A lot of great information how to get to the right place. Alan A, Newberry Park , CA

We really like the conversational tone. The subject is so serious...it is so nice to read something that is not too technical, not condescending. '...this was written for me.' Lindsay F, Los Angeles, CA

What physicians are saying about
Brain Tumors-Leaving the Garden of Eden

Informative...written with ...a nice blend of compassion... providing sensitive information and respecting the patients' intelligence.
Dr Maria Bishop, Arizona Cancer Center, Tucson

Packed with practical information and inspiring stories from patients and families who have "been there,..."

Like a compass in the wilderness, ... a user-friendly tool for plotting an early course through the uncertainties of diagnosis and treatment of a brain tumor. Dr. Henry Friedman & Bebe Guill, Tug Mcgraw Neuro-Oncology Quality Of Life Center, Duke University, Durham, NC (See page 396 for additional comments from professionals).